ALLERGIES

ALLERGIES

Dr D G Delvin

MB BS LRCP MRCS DOBST
RCOG DCH FPA CERT
MRCGP DIP VEN
MFFP

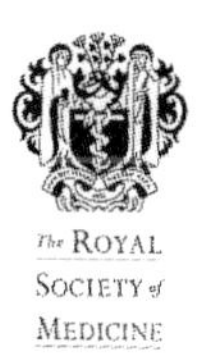

The Royal
Society of
Medicine

SUNBURST BOOKS

Editorial Advisor

DR KATHARINE A ORTON
MB BS MRCGP
DCH DRCOG

ACKNOWLEDGEMENT

I should like to express my special thanks to Dr Katharine Orton for her advice in the planning of this book.

This edition first published in 1995 by
Sunburst Books, Deacon House,
65 Old Church Street, London SW3 5BS.

ISBN 1 85778 161 9

Printed and bound in China

INTRODUCTION

Many millions of people worldwide have allergies – some trivial, some very serious. And for reasons we don't entirely understand, the number of people with allergies is increasing.

In fact, there is a lot we don't understand about allergy. It is a confusing subject and there is still no completely clear and unambiguous definition of what an allergy actually is. However, if you read the entry on ***Allergy*** on page 14, it should give you a much better understanding of the subject.

Please bear in mind that allergy has no connection with dislike, nor is allergy the same thing as sensitivity. You can be unusually sensitive to colds, criticism, hot weather or even to certain drugs, but this does not mean that your body produces an allergic reaction to these things.

Good luck with defeating your personal allergy. But before you dip into this book, do please read the health warning overleaf.

Dr David Delvin

HEALTH WARNING

No book can take the place of a doctor, so always be guided by your general practitioner or specialist. And please bear the following points in mind while reading this book:

* Medical science changes rapidly, so always ask your doctor for the most up-to-date information

* Knowledge about drugs changes very fast indeed, and many of the drugs listed in this book will eventually turn out to have side-effects which we do not yet know about

* This book lists only a selection of the possible side-effects of the drugs mentioned. For further information, ask your doctor or pharmacist

* Always remember that drugs can interact with each other, and seek the latest professional advice

* If you are pregnant or breast-feeding, do not take any drugs at all unless your doctor says it is safe to do so

ADDITIVES

These days an enormous variety of chemicals is added to our food. Unfortunately, some people develop adverse reactions to these additives.

It is often difficult to find out whether a symptom is really caused by a food additive. Even if it *is*, it may not necessarily be a true allergic reaction. If you read the section on **Allergy**, you will see that there are many symptoms that are caused by external agents but which are not actually allergies. They are just 'bad reactions'.

Additives fall into the following main groups:

Colourings These are added to your food to make it look better, for commercial purposes

Preservatives Put in food to prevent germ growth and give the product a longer shelf-life

Flavourings Added to try and make the food more tasty or to disguise less pleasant tastes

Sweeteners These include sugar (sucrose), and are added to give the product a sweeter taste. Few people realise just how much sweetening is added to tinned and packet goods. For instance, the average can of baked beans contains 25 grammes of sugar – five heaped teaspoonfuls.

Anti-oxidants Some foods go darker or look less attractive when they are exposed to oxygen in the air (an obvious example is the way an apple turns brown once it has been bitten into).

Antioxidants are chemicals that prevent this change from occurring, for commercial purposes.

Bleaches Chemicals that whiten food (eg bread) to make it more attractive to some people

E NUMBERS Strangely, in much of the world the majority of food additives are not listed on the packaging. In many countries, several thousands of these additives are widely used but only a few hundred are named on the labelling. This makes it very difficult to decide whether or not a person's symptoms are caused by an additive.

In the European Union (EU) only a minority of additives are listed on food labelling. These are the 'E number' additives ('E' stands for Europe).

E number additives have been approved by the EU, but that does not mean that they cannot cause allergies or other bad reactions.

If you or one of your family has odd symptoms – or perhaps worsening of an allergy – it is worth considering whether excluding certain E number additives from the diet might be helpful. However, in a long career as a doctor, I have not yet seen an allergic person whose condition has been significantly improved by avoiding these additives.

Nonetheless, because there is so much interest in this subject (particularly among parents), some of the E numbers which are commonly alleged to cause health problems are listed below:

Colouring additives (E100 to E180) In this group, interest has centred on the following:-

* **E102** (Tartrazine) A yellow dye, said to provoke asthma and hyperactive behaviour

* **E123** (Amaranth) An azo dye, also said to provoke hyperactivity and asthma

* **E150** (Caramel) Colourant used in biscuits, 'junk' foods, etc. Said to provoke hyperactivity

Preservatives (E200 to E297) In this group, interest has centred on:

* **E210 to 219** (Various benzoates) Said to cause asthma and skin problems

* **E222** (Sodium bisulphite) This preservative is said to cause asthma

* **E252** (Potassium nitrate) Said to cause skin problems and hyperactivity

ADRENALINE

An enormously useful anti-allergy drug, known in the United States and some other countries as epinephrine or by the trade name Adrenalin. It is particularly valuable in severe attacks of asthma (*see* **Asthma**), because it widens the air passages that lead to the lungs – a potentailly life-saving property. Unfortunately, adrenaline cannot be taken by mouth because it is destroyed by stomach juices, so it has to be given by injection. The injection must be given with great care, because even a small overdose of adrenaline can be dangerous.

AIR POLLUTION

It is widely believed that the increase in air pollution in recent years is at least partly responsible for the increased occurrence of asthma and other allergies. However, the latest research suggests that allergic illnesses have become more common in relatively unpolluted areas of the world, as well as in polluted ones.

But what is undisputed is that air pollutants do cause considerable difficulties for many people who have allergies. There is little evidence that people are allergic to the air pollutants – the problem is that these pollutants aggravate the symptoms. In particular, they can cause intense breathing difficulties for asthmatics because they irritate the air passages. People with hay fever and other nasal allergies may also find that pollution makes their symptoms worse, and causes runny eyes and sneezing.

THE POLLUTANTS Air pollutants vary in different parts of the world, but the commonest include:

Cigarette smoke Because this is not produced by an industrial process, it is often forgotten that it is a major air pollutant, especially in the home. It is a particular nuisance to people with asthma, hay fever and other nasal allergies.

Carbon monoxide Produced by combustion, and by vehicle exhausts. It is thought to play a part in causing heart disease.

CFCs Produced by aerosols and the chemical industry. Irritate the respiratory tract and eyes.

Formaldehyde Produced by industry and vehicle exhausts. Irritates the lungs.

Hydrogen sulphide Produced by refineries and sewage. Irritates the eyes and nose.

Methane Produced by sewage, rotting waste, and cattle (flatus). Irritates the lungs.

Nitric acid Produced by the action of light on nitrogen dioxide. Irritates the lungs.

Nitrogen oxides Produced by combustion and vehicle exhausts. Irritates the air passages.

Ozone Produced by the effect of light on nitrogen oxides. Irritates the eyes and lungs.

Sulphur dioxide Produced by combustion and smelting. Irritates the eyes and lungs.

In general, if you suffer from a respiratory allergy such as asthma, it is a good idea to keep as far away as possible from polluted air. Often, a simple measure such as going to the relatively unpolluted air of the countryside or seaside will improve symptoms.

ALLERGENS

An allergen is anything which is capable of provoking an allergy (*see* **Allergy**). Some common allergens include:

* pollen
* mould
* house dust mites (or their droppings)
* hairs of cats, horses and other pets
* dander (shed skin cells) from animals
* certain foods
* certain drugs
* sticking plaster
* detergents

An allergen has no effect on a person who does not have allergic tendencies, but if you have got a tendency towards allergy, then exposure to an allergen can cause you a lot of trouble. This will not happen the first time you are exposed to it. Indeed, you may have many exposures without any problems, but eventually, your body may make antibodies to the allergen (*see* **Antibodies**).

If this happens, the next time you are exposed to the allergen, there will be a violent reaction between it and your antibodies, which will make your cells release the powerful chemicals that give you the symptoms of an allergy.

Unless you get treatment, all future exposures to the allergen will have a similar effect. However, there is sometimes a tendency for the body's responses to an allergen to change as time goes by, and a person with a life-long allergy may find that as the years pass she is no longer affected.

ALLERGIC RHINITIS

Any of the group of conditions in which the nose becomes inflamed as a result of an allergy. Rhinitis just means inflammation of the nose. Conditions in this group include:

* hay fever (*see* **Hay fever**)
* dust mite allergy (*see* **House dust**)
* perennial rhinitis – a condition in which hay fever-type symptoms occur on almost every day of the year (*see* **Perennial rhinitis**)

Treatment for all types of rhinitis includes:

* avoiding the allergen (provoking factor)
* anti-histamine drugs (*see* **Anti-histamines**)
* using Intal-type drugs (*see* **Cromoglycate**)
* using nasal steroids (*see* **Steroids**)
* using desensitisation (*see* **Desensitisation**)
  For a full description of treatment of rhinitis *see* **Hay fever**

ALLERGY

An allergy is a mistaken defence reaction by the body; this is meant to protect you, but in fact it is very troublesome. Most people do not have any allergic tendencies but the minority proportion of those who do suffer is increasing, although the reason for this growth is presently unknown.

If you do have an allergic tendency, from time to time something – whether it be pollen, a drug or a certain food – comes along that makes your body's protective system say: 'Hello, this is something foreign'.

Your protective system – which is actually called the immune system – doesn't take any action there and then, so you will be unaware of any problem. The immune system just makes a careful note of the characteristics of the 'foreign invader'. But next time the invader – which is medically known as an allergen – turns up, your immune system says: 'Here's that enemy again. Let's defend ourself'. You can clearly see that this is quite different from just being unusually vulnerable or sensitive to an external influence.

Unfortunately, the defence turns out to be a massively over-the-top reaction known as the allergic response. The defenders are called antibodies, and were formed by your body in response to the first visit of the foreign invader. They go completely wild, and start attacking your own cells. In particular, they attack cells called mast cells, which are found in your nose, lungs and skin, and some other tissues as well. When the mast cells are broken open by the assault, they release all sorts of harmful chemicals – but especially one called histamine.

Histamine causes inflammation wherever is it released. Inflammation is characterised by the following problems:

* redness
* swelling
* discomfort
* itching
* leakage of fluid from blood vessels

The effect this has on you depends on precisely where this violent reaction occurs. Some of the possibilities are as follows:

* If it happens in your nose, you'll get some form of rhinitis (*see* **Rhinitis**), such as hay fever

* If it happens in your lungs and the air passages leading to them, you'll get an attack of asthma (*see* **Asthma**)

* If it happens in your skin, you'll get some form of rash or eruption – for instance, eczema (*see* **Eczema**) or urticaria (*see* **Urticaria**)

You can see that the effects of an allergic reaction can be very diverse, but they usually involve the release of histamine. This is why drugs called anti-histamines, which oppose its action, are so often useful in cases of allergy (*see* **Anti-histamines**).

Why do only some people get allergies? This is a very difficult question to answer. It has been known for a long time that allergy tends to run in families – though it may not always be the same allergy. For instance, a parent may have hay fever or asthma, and their son may have eczema.

So it does seem as though there may be some hereditary factor which makes people vulnerable to allergy. On the other hand, there are plenty of men and women who develop allergies even though there does not appear to be a history of allergic disorders in their families.

One important point is that people who are liable to allergies tend to have a higher than normal level of the antibody immunoglobulin E (IgE).

IgE – pronounced as the letters i, g, e – is found only in very low levels in the blood of non-allergic children. But it is thought that if a newborn baby has a substantial amount of this antibody in his blood, he will be more likely to have allergic problems later in life (*see also* **IgE**).

Rare types of allergy Up until now we have been talking about the common types of allergy which occur in everyday conditions familiar to most people – things such as asthma, hay fever and eczema. As we have seen, these occur because antibodies (usually IgE) attack body cells, and cause the release of histamine and other harmful chemicals. Doctors call this a type one allergy.

There are other types of allergy as well. However, unless you have been told that your allergic condition is one of them, you don't need to read the next three paragraphs.

Type two allergies In these, the allergen attaches itself to certain types of body cell before being attacked by antibodies. Some very unusual kinds of anaemia ('weak blood') are caused in this way.

Type three allergies These are very complicated reactions, in which the allergen forms clumps of material in the blood, along with antibodies (not IgE, but one called IgG) and a natural product called complement. It is possible that this kind of reaction is involved in some food allergies. It certainly occurs in an uncommon condition called serum sickness (*see* **Serum Sickness**).

Type four allergies Unlike other allergies, these do not involve antibodies, only a certain type of white blood cells called thymus-derived lymphocytes. These reactions are much slower than 'ordinary' allergies, and may take up to four days to develop. They include contact dermatitis (*see* **Dermatitis**).

As you can see, allergy is an immensely complicated subject and, there is an awful lot that doctors don't yet know about it. Without doubt, we shall find out a great deal more over the next few years.

One mystery which may or may not be resolved is this: why are humans so prone to allergy? After all, animals don't seem to suffer from it in the same extraordinary way.

A possible answer could be that allergy somehow confers some benefit on the human race. That may seem unlikely, but scientists have recently shown that IgE (which, as we've seen, is present at a high level in the blood of allergic people) is useful in defending humans against parasite infections, which have plagued them, especially in the tropics, for many thousands of years.

Furthermore, US biologists have suggested that allergic responses such as streaming eyes and coughing can actually help people get rid of toxins which enter their eyes or air passages.

Finally, it has even been suggested recently that allergic people are less likely to develop cancer than non-allergic people are. However, this fascinating theory remains very much unproven.

ANAPHYLAXIS

Pronounced 'Anna-fill-AXE-iss', this is a severe allergic reaction in which the person collapses and may even die. Fortunately, it is very rare.

It used to happen more frequently in the days when people were given blood serum, taken from horses, to protect them against infection. Nowadays, it is much more likely to be provoked by one of the following things:

* penicillin, and sometimes other antibiotics
* bee stings, and occasionally wasp stings
* certain foods, especially nuts (*see* **Nuts)**
* injected X-ray dyes

Anaphylaxis is a dramatic condition, which comes on very rapidly – and usually very soon after exposure to the allergen. Symptoms may include:

* collapse
* striking rash
* abdominal pain, diarrhoea and/or vomiting
* severe breathing problems
* swelling of the throat and mouth

Fast action is essential, or death may occur. Get the victim to a doctor or hospital straight away. Be prepared to give the kiss of life and/or heart massage. People who have had previous episodes of anaphylaxis should carry a warning Medic-Alert bracelet and an anti-histamine pill. There is also a case for obtaining an adrenaline injection kit from your doctor (*see* **Adrenaline**).

ANGIO-OEDEMA

This is a severe type of allergic reaction, in which the eyelids. face and throat swell up – so there can be serious difficulty with breathing. Swelling may also occur in the fingers and joints.

Angio-oedema is closely related to urticaria (*see* **Urticaria**), a condition which affects the skin. Angio-oedema affects other tissues. Some people have both conditions.

If an attack occurs, get the patient to a doctor or a hospital as quickly as possible.

Angio-oedema used to be known as 'angio-neurotic oedema', but this misleading name has now been abandoned. The condition has nothing whatever to do with neurosis.

ANIMAL ALLERGIES

Many people are allergic to certain animals – or rather, to material from animals such as hair or dander (shed skin cells). Symptoms include:

* rashes
* sneezing
* runny nose and eyes
* wheezing

If you suspect an animal allergy, do ***not*** just get rid of your pet. Instead, go to your doctor, discuss the symptoms, and have the necessary tests done to try to establish the precise cause of the allergy.

If it transpires that the person really is allergic to a particular type of animal, then clearly it is best to avoid contact in future if at all possible. Anti-allergy medication such as anti-histamines may also be helpful. Unfortunately, desensitisation injections (*see* **Desensitisation**) have not proved very effective.

ANTIBODIES

Antibodies are formed by the body in response to any challenge from an 'invader'. The invader is called an antigen (*see* **Antigens**, below), and it is the antibody's job to combine with it and so make it harmless.

Unfortunately, in allergies, antibodies are formed in response to some harmless challenge from (say) pollen, and the antibodies then create havoc by attacking the body's own cells.

This attack releases histamine and other toxic chemicals and you immediately develop the symptoms of an allergy (*see also* **Allergy**).

ANTIGENS

Antigens are foreign 'invaders' which provoke the body to produce antibodies against them (*see* **Antibodies**).

In cases of allergy, the antigens are referred to as allergens (*see* **Allergens**).

Many antigens are proteins. Those which are not proteins achieve 'protein status' by combining with one of the body's own proteins.

ANTI-HISTAMINES

These are drugs which are very useful in combating the symptoms of allergy. They cannot cure the condition, but they can make it very much more bearable.

How do they do it? If you read the entry on **Allergy**, you will see that an allergic reaction usually involves the release of a chemical called histamine from the body's cells. This chemical is extremely troublesome, because it causes the inflammatory symptoms which make allergy such a nuisance.

Anti-histamines are drugs that are chemically related to histamine, but which have the property of blocking its effects. They are particularly useful in conditions such as hay fever (and other forms of rhinitis – nose inflammation) and urticaria, but are not of real use in asthma.

For many years, the main problem with anti-histamines was that they were also sedatives. Indeed, they sedate the brain so much that some of them are used as sleeping pills. This made it dangerous to take anti-histamines if you were going to drive or operate machinery, and it also made school work quite difficult for some children. This was most unfortunate in certain countries where the hay fever season coincided with the exam season.

All that began to change in the 1980s when the new non-sedative anti-histamines were introduced. Although it cannot be guaranteed that these non-sedative drugs will not cause drowsiness or slow reactions, they are certainly very much less likely to do so than the older types of anti-histamine.

However, they do have their own side-effects, which you should be aware of – especially as they are now sold widely over-the-counter – that is, without a doctor's prescription. Some of these side-effects are detailed below.

The principal anti-histamines used against allergy today are as follows:

SEDATIVE ANTI-HISTAMINES Please note that although these drugs might be considered old-fashioned and have a tendency to cause drowsiness, they are still favoured by a lot of people who have allergies.

You must ***not*** take them if you are going to drive a vehicle. Operating machinery could also be dangerous, and there are circumstances where it would clearly be most unwise to use computers or delicate machinery, or indeed make any important decisions.

Under no circumstances should you take any alcohol while on any of the following sedative anti-histamines:

* Atarax (hydroxyzine)
* Daneral SA (pheniramine)
* Dimotane (brompheniramine)
* Phenergan (promethazine)
* Piriton (chlorpheniramine)
* Primalan (mecuitazine)
* Tavegil (clemastine)
* Ucerax (hydroxyzine)
* Vallergen (trimeprazine)

NON-SEDATIVE ANTI-HISTAMINES Even these can have some sedating properties, so I recommend that you do not take alcohol or any other sedative drug with them. If you feel the slightest bit drowsy, do not drive, and let your doctor know that you have experienced this effect. There are also other possible side-effects associated with certain drugs:

* Clarityn (loratidine) – can cause tiredness, vomiting and headache
* Hismanal (astemizole) – can cause weight gain and occasionally heart problems; including palpitations and irregular beating

* Semprex (acrivastine) – drowsiness is possible but uncommon

* Triludan (terfenadine) – can cause headache, rashes, tummy upset or sweating, and occasionally heart problems; do not exceed the stated dose, and do not take with anti-fungal drugs, certain antibiotics or astemizole. Ask your doctor or chemist for further advice

* Zirtek (cetrizine) – can cause headache, dizziness, tummy upset or agitation

Other side-effects of anti-histamines Although anti-histamines are so useful against allergy, they can sometimes have rare side-effects, and you should be guided by your own doctor about these. Such effects may include dryness of the mouth, difficulty in passing urine, blurry vision and odd skin reactions when exposed to sunlight. Avoid these drugs if you are breast-feeding.

ANTI-HISTAMINES ON THE SKIN Anti-histamines in cream or ointment form are often sold over-the counter for application to areas of inflamed skin (often in cases where the inflammation has not even been caused by allergy). In general, dermatologists are against using anti-histamines in this way, as they can sometimes cause severe sensitivity reactions.

ASTHMA

Asthma is one of the most common of all allergic disorders. In many Western countries it now affects about five per cent (one in 20) of the population, and this proportion is increasing.

The reasons for this increase are not clear. It is possible that doctors are simply diagnosing the disease more often then they used to. Another factor may be the increase in the amount of atmospheric pollution in recent years, though it is believed that asthma is also increasing in relatively unpolluted regions of the world.

WHAT IS ASTHMA? It is a narrowing of the air passages (tubes) which carry air into the lungs. This narrowing is not present all the time, but when it happens the air tubes contract down with the result that the victim finds it very difficult to draw air into her body, and to blow it out again.

Asthma – sometimes known as bronchial asthma – is therefore characterised by attacks of breathlessness, accompanied by wheezing. Often, this sound can be heard several metres away from the patient.

The air tubes get narrower for several reasons:

* The muscle in the walls of the tubes contracts

* The lining of the tubes becomes swollen, narrowing the space available for air

* Sticky secretions (mucus) pour out into the tubes and help to block them up

> The result is that it becomes much harder for the sufferer to breathe. Air becomes trapped in the lungs, and the sufferer may find that she cannot clear out the sticky mucus by coughing it up.

It is vitally important to realise that this narrowing of the tubes is potentially serious. If they are badly blocked, death may easily result.

Many asthmatics die each year, and in many cases their deaths are needless. Fast medical attention can often save the sufferer, so never hesitate to seek immediate medical help if someone has a bad attack of asthma.

CAUSES It used to be said that asthma was caused by three factors:

* allergy
* infection
* psychological strain

These days, most doctors would say that the psychological aspect is a very minor one. It is possible that when people get very worked up they bring on an attack of asthma, but this is not a factor of great significance.

Asthma usually begins either in childhood or in the middle part of life, with boys being affected more often than girls.

Many cases are caused by allergy, and asthma

attacks may also be provoked or made worse by a chest infection.

Early onset asthma In asthma that begins in childhood or early adult life, there is almost invariably a strong allergic component. These youngsters often come from families in which allergy is common. Frequently, mumor dad may have hay fever, eczema or maybe asthma itself.

Children and teenagers who have an asthmatic tendency will usually have high blood levels of a substance called IgE (*see* **IgE**), which is an indicator of an allergic tendency. Skin sensitivity tests on these youngsters will frequently show that they are allergic to quite a wide range of things, such as feathers, wool, pollen and dust mites.

Unfortunately, it is not often possible to say with any certainty that it is one particular thing that is causing the asthmatic attacks. However, parents sometimes find that taking a child away from her usual environment (even, perhaps, sending her to boarding school if finances permit) can lead to an improvement in her condition, which suggests that the move has got her away from the substances that were causing the trouble. Nevertheless, I do not suggest that you move house or send your child away to boarding school unless your pediatrician says that there is some extremely good reason for doing so.

Some asthmatic children also have eczema and/or hay fever and/or skin allergies, which reinforces the point that they are highly allergic individuals.

Late onset asthma This is the type that comes on in the middle years of life. The link with allergy in these patients is nothing like as clear, and we really have little idea why people in their 30s, 40s and 50s sometimes get asthma.

AGGRAVATING FACTORS It is most important to realise that asthma may be aggravated by all sorts of factors. These include:

* Cigarette smoking It is complete lunacy for an asthmatic to smoke. Parents of asthmatic children should try their hardest not to smoke – or at least, only do it far away from the child. People with asthma should keep out of smoky rooms, and always make sure to travel in non-smoking compartments. They should also ask to be seated in non-smoking areas in restaurants
* Air pollution (*see* **Air Pollution**)
* Exercise Though a certain amount of exercise is usually good for asthmatics, some children find that their attacks are actually brought on by exertion
* Breathing in cold air There is much to be said for wearing a scarf across your mouth in cold weather if you suffer from asthma
* Respiratory infections Asthma patients should always visit their doctor for

treatment immediately if they develop a cough

* Stress As I have already mentioned, psychological stress is not now rated as an important factor in provoking asthma attacks. Nonetheless, if you have asthma it is a good idea to try and avoid anxiety and strain, and to get plenty of rest.

SYMPTOMS The main symptoms of an asthma attack are as follows:

* wheezing
* breathlessness
* tightness in the chest
* cough
* rapid heartbeat
* occasionally, blueness of the face in the case of a severe attack

Attacks may last anything from a few minutes to several hours. Typically, the victim sits upright, holding her shoulder muscles taut in an attempt to aid the fight for breath.

Between attacks, asthma patients may be perfectly well, though some have a permanent slight wheeze.

TESTS If you develop asthma, it is very important that you have certain investigations to help assess your condition, and to monitor it as time goes by. These investigations include:

* Lung function tests These are tests in which you to blow into various pieces of apparatus. You should make yourself thoroughly familiar with one particular lung function test, which is called 'peak flow' or 'peak expiratory flow' (PEF). There is a strong case for doing this test regularly and frequently, and many asthmatic people now have their own peak flow meters, and keep a chart of their own readings. This is extremely helpful, because the chart can help show whether your asthma is going into a phase that requires help in the form of extra medication

* Chest X-ray

* Blood gas tests These are vital in the event of a bad attack of asthma. A sample of blood is taken from an artery, in order to find out the pressure of oxygen and carbon dioxide (CO_2) in the blood

* Skin tests These are done by pricking various olutions through the skin (*see* **Prick tests**) to try and see if you are allergic to them. Unfortunately, the information obtained isn't usually of great use in helping the person to avoid factors which provoke attacks

TREATMENT The treatment of asthma has made great strides in recent years, but even so asthmatics do not always get the best treatment fast enough. If an attack does not seem to be clearing up rapidly, never hesitate to get medical help.

There are various aspects of treatment and of trying to prevent the occurrence of an attack:

Leading a sensible life As already mentioned, asthmatic people should avoid cigarette smoke and other forms of air pollution. They should also avoid breathing in very cold air. A child who has exercise-induced asthma should be excused from energetic school sports. If an allergen (provoking factor) has been identified, keep away from it.

However, asthmatic people should not let themselves be molly-coddled, and should lead as full a life as possible.

Desensitisation (hyposensitisation) In the past, there were great hopes for the technique of desensitising an allergic person by injecting her with tiny amounts of whatever the allergen (*see* **Allergen**). This therapy was particularly popular in the United States.

Unfortunately, however, it does not work very well in asthma. Furthermore, so many people have had serious side-effects (eg life-threatening collapse) from the injections that they have been virtually abandoned in many parts of the world.

Clinical ecologists (*see* **Clinical ecology**) do still use desensitisation extensively, though in addition to injections into the skin they often give drops under the tongue. This is certainly very safe, but orthodox doctors who specialise in allergy are dubious about its benefits.

Drugs A wealth of drugs is now available for controlling and treating asthma, but all of them must be used with great care. Always bear in mind that an overdose may be very dangerous. Drugs in use today fall into the following groups:

* Sodium cromoglycate (Intal) and ketotifen (Zaditen). Intal – sucked into the lungs from a special inhaler – has been available for nearly 30 years as a preventer of asthma attacks. It must be taken regularly and long-term, to help keep attacks away. It is of no use in an actual attack. Zaditen – which, though taken by mouth, works in a similar way to Intal – has the disadvantage of causing drowsiness

* Bronchodilators. This word means 'drugs which widen the air passages'. There are four basic types:

1 **Beta$_2$ stimulants** These include salbutamol (Ventolin), terbutaline (Bricanyl), fenoterol (Berotec), rimiterol (Pulmadil) and salmeterol (Serevent). Serevent should not be used in an actual attack, because it is too slow-acting. The drugs are generally given in pressurised aerosols, and it is vital that the sufferer knows the correct technique for using these devices.

2 **Anticholinergics** These drugs tend to be used more in chronic bronchitis, but have some value in asthma. They include oxitropium

(Oxivent) and ipratropium (Atrovent). They are usually given by aerosol.

3 Theophylline-type Theophylline is an old remedy, related to caffeine (the drug in coffee and tea). Members of this group still have some value in widening the air passages. They include theophylline itself (Nuelin), choline theophyllinate (Choledyl) and aminophylline (Pecram, Phyllocontin).

4 Compound preparations These contain combinations of various drugs. They include Duovent and Franol.

* Steroids. These drugs are extremely valuable and can be life-saving in asthma. If your physician agrees, it is often worth having a small supply of oral steroid tablets at home in case of emergency. For further details and warnings, *see* **Steroids**

SPECIAL DEVICES FOR ASTHMA PATIENTS A number of devices that can help asthmatic people by administering their drugs more effectively have been developed in recent years. They include:

* The Spinhaler. A 'turbo' device for the administration of Intal powder from a capsule by inhalation

* Spacers. These often look rather like large balloons. They provide a space between an inhaler and the patient's mouth, to slow down the aerosol particles, and thus

increase their chances of getting all the way down to the lungs

* Nebulisers. These turn a solution of an anti-asthma drug into an aerosol, which allows a higher dose of the drug to be inhaled. There are circumstances where this is desirable, but there are also many times when it is *not* a good idea to give yourself a higher dose. So please be advised by your doctor

ATOPY

This word is often found in books and articles about asthma, eczema and related conditions. It is just another word for allergy, and the word 'atopic' similarly just means 'allergic'.

BEE STINGS

For most people, bee stings are unpleasant and painful, but the problem will soon be over if you use sensible first aid measures – carefully remove the sting with tweezers; apply a cold compress; if necessary, take a pain-killer such as aspirin or paracetamol.

But in some allergic people, a bee sting may cause the frightening collapse called anaphylactic shock or anaphylaxis (*see* **Anaphylaxis**). If someone suddenly feels very ill after a bee sting, you must get them to a doctor or hospital *at once.* Be prepared to give the kiss of life and heart massage if necessary.

If you are an allergic person who has previously

had a serious reaction to a bee sting, you need to take great care to avoid such stings in the future because they could put your life at risk.

Therefore, you should avoid bees. When they are around, take great care where you put your hands. Don't wear scent or aftershave when you are out in the open air. Be careful when drinking outside – the glass might have a bee on the rim. If a bee approaches you do ***not*** flap at it. They usually will not bother you, and will normally go away if you keep still. If your physician agrees, it may be worth having an adrenaline injection kit available in case of a sting.

Desensitisation against bee stings is possible, but time-consuming.

BREAST-FEEDING AND ALLERGY

Breast-feeding is by far the best thing for human babies. Among its many benefits is the fact that babies who are breast-fed have a lower chance of being allergic than those who are bottle-fed.

In particular, it has been shown that breast-fed babies are much less likely to get eczema. This is not really surprising. Bottle milk is, after all, cow's milk, so it contains all sorts of proteins which are fine for calves, but which are 'foreign' to the immune system of a human baby.
So do try and breast-feed your children, especially if there is a tendency to allergy in your family (*see also* **Cows milk allergy**).

CLINICAL ECOLOGY

A form of alternative medicine which is currently extremely popular in America, Australia, New Zealand and Britain. It is practised by doctors who claim to be able to use it to treat allergies. Orthodox medicine views these claims with great cynicism.

Nonetheless, the basic principle of clinical ecology – that the body can easily become allergic, or sensitive, to the many environmental factors we are exposed to today – is an attractive one. Clinical ecologists are particularly interested in the idea that a lot of people's symptoms are actually caused by allergies to a particular type of food.

Some doctors who work in this field have promoted the idea that there are people who are sensitive to practically everything they come into contact with (*see* **Total allergy syndrome**). However, there are virtually no allergy experts who take this idea seriously.

Clinical ecologists carry out allergy tests such as the RAST (or Radio Allergo Sorbent Test), the auricular cardiac reflex (ACR) and the cytotoxicity test, which are not at present widely accepted by orthodox allergists.

The methods of treatment used include exclusion diets, in which certain items of food are omitted from the diet to see if the symptoms improve, and a form of desensitisation (*see under* **Desensitisation**) in which small amounts of the suspected allergen are given to the patient – usually as drops under the tongue.

CONDOM ALLERGY

This is not uncommon, and may give either partner sore and/or itching genitals. The manufacturers state that it is not usually rubber causing the problem, but chemical additives. They offer low allergy brands which contain hardly any of these additives.

If the problem persists, an alternative is to use 'Fourex' – condoms which are designed to avoid any possible rubber or chemical allergy because they are made from lambs' intestines. However, some couples find these quite unacceptable on ethical or aesthetic grounds.

In such cases, the only answer is to switch to another method of contraception – for instance, the female condom (Femidom), which is not made of rubber.

CONJUNCTIVITIS

This means inflammation of the transparent membrane which covers the front of the eye. Symptoms may include:

* itching
* soreness
* watering

Conjunctivitis is often caused by allergy. This may be the result of medication (drops or ointment) put into the eye, or to foreign matter, such as pollen, which has drifted into it.

If you find that using a particular medication causes conjunctivitis, you should stop using it immediately, and consult your doctor. The same applies if you find that contact lens fluids give you a pink, runny eye, or if cosmetics cause the same problem.

Conjunctivitis caused by pollen or other foreign airborne material is usually associated with allergic rhinitis (*see* **Allergic rhinitis**).

Treatment for the eyes is described in the section on **Hay fever**.

CONTACT DERMATITIS

Dermatitis means inflammation of the skin and, as the name suggests, contact dermatitis is caused by contact between the skin and some external agent.

Many cases of contact dermatitis are *not* caused by allergy – even a non-allergic person's skin will become inflamed if it comes into contact with something irritant.

However, very often contact dermatitis *is* the result of an allergic reaction. In some instances, this occurs very rapidly; in others, it takes a few days to develop.

The appearance of the skin in contact dermatitis may well provide the diagnosis because the area of inflammation is often the same shape as whatever was in contact with it. Thus, the back of a watch will produce a disc-shaped eruption on the wrist. The skin will be angry-looking, red (in fair-skinned people) and often weeping. Usually it will itch.

Some things which commonly cause dermatitis include the following:

* nickel – a metal found in jewellery, coins, and clothes fasteners
* sticking plaster
* chemicals in shoes and gloves
* deodorants – the eruption will be in the armpit only
* shampoos, hair sprays, cosmetics
* lanolin (sheep's wool fat)
* plants – especially poison ivy in the United States

There are countless others. If the cause is not immediately obvious, your doctor may well suggest patch tests on your skin to identify the allergen. Unfortunately, desensitisation is not usually a possibility, and the best 'treatment' is to keep well away from the offending material in future. Unexpected flare-ups can be treated with steroid ointments or creams.

COSMETICS

These are a common cause of contact dermatitis (*see* **Contact dermatitis**).

If you suddenly develop a skin rash or an eye irritation after changing to a new brand of make-up, there is a high chance that this product is responsible. You should stop using it at once, and check with your doctor. If she agrees, it may be possible to do a simple allergy test by taping a small amount of the new make-up to your forearm and seeing if there is any reaction.

If you are allergic to a brand, the only solution is to discontinue its use. It is not possible to use desensitisation (*see* **Desensitisation**).

It is most unlikely that you could have any legal claim against the manufacturers. Your only hope of success in court would be if you could prove that they had been in some way negligent – for example, if you could show that so many women had complained about the brand that they should have printed a warning about possible reactions.

COW'S MILK ALLERGY

As explained in the section on ***Breast-feeding and allergy***, cow's milk contains proteins which are ideal for calves, but which are not 'designed' for humans.

It is not surprising, therefore, that a proportion of children – believed to be about one in a hundred – are allergic to cow's milk. There is a strong family tendency to this allergy, and boys are affected more often than girls.

Symptoms which show that a child suffers from

this allergy usually appear in the first year of life. These symptoms may include:

* skin rashes (including eczema)
* diarrhoea and vomiting
* failure to put on weight
* wheezing
* feeling miserable and crying a lot
* snuffling

In the old days, these babies went completely undiagnosed. Most did eventually recover from their allergy, but at considerable cost to their well-being.

It is now recognised that It is far better to try and diagnose the problem early. If you suspect that your baby has an allergy to cow's milk, talk it over with your GP. She may suggest a diet which contains no cow's milk (perhaps containing soya milk instead), but this should be carefully worked out with a dietitian or other qualified professional.

Note: Cow's milk allergy has no connection with the milk-sugar (lactose) intolerance often seen in Asian children. This is not an allergic reaction.

CROMOGLYCATE

A very useful anti-allergy drug which was first discovered in the mid-1960s. Its full name is disodium cromoglycate and it is marketed under various trade names, such as Intal, lomusol and Rynacrom.

It works by stabilising certain body cells that are attacked by the allergic reaction. It must be taken long-term – in other words, as a protectant. It is never of any use in treating an actual attack of an allergy.

Further details of the use of cromoglycate are found in the sections on ***Asthma***, ***Hay fever*** and ***Food allergies***.

DERMATITIS

The word dermatitis simply means inflammation of the skin.

Unfortunately, there is still a great deal of muddle and confusion in the way that skin disorders are named, and in many parts of the world, dermatitis simply means eczema (*see* **Eczema**).

Dermatitis caused by physical contact with something is called contact dermatitis (*see* **Contact dermatitis**).

DESENSITISATION

This is a process whereby a person can sometimes be cured of his allergy (or at least have it made much milder). It is done by giving repeated injections of very small amounts of the material which has been causing the problem.

It is not at all clear why desensitisation – also known as hyposensitisation – works, but the fact is that it can be highly effective.

However, in recent years it has become much less popular in many parts of the world, as a result of the fact that the injections themselves can sometimes cause severe, and even fatal, reactions.

Desensitisation against bee and wasp stings is still used, because people who are allergic to these stings are at risk of serious illness (or even death) from anaphylaxis (*see* **Anaphylaxis**). The injections must only be given in premises where full resuscitation facilities are available, in case of collapse.

Practitioners of clinical ecology carry out a totally different type of attempted desensitisation. Most orthodox doctors do not believe that this works (*see* **Clinical ecology**).

DETERGENTS

Detergents are a common cause of allergies – especially skin allergies of the contact dermatitis type (*see* **Contact dermatitis**). Biological washing powders may cause more trouble than others.

It is usually the person who is doing the washing who tends to develop an allergic reaction to a detergent, but people who are involved in the manufacturing process are also at risk, and sometimes the wearer of an item of clothing may develop a skin reaction if detergent has been left in the clothes.

If you suspect a detergent allergy, then the obvious thing to do is to change your detergent and see what happens. If in doubt, your doctor may be willing to set up a simple skin test to see if you really are allergic to a particular brand.

Desensitisation against detergents is not practicable, so the only remedy for this condition is to avoid the offending detergent.

DIET (EXCLUSION)

In cases of possible food allergy *(see **Food allergies**)*, it is worth trying an exclusion or elimination diet. However, my advice is not to try this without advice from a doctor or dietitian.

Certainly, no baby or child should be put on an exclusion diet without the careful supervision of a qualified health professional. There have been cases where parents have unwisely put their children on dietary regimes which have been deficient in vital nutrients.

The general idea of an exclusion diet is to cut out the food that you suspect is causing trouble and see if symptoms disappear. If they do then the food should be reintroduced a few days later to see if the symptoms return.

There are more scientific ways of doing dietary testing. For instance a medical specialist might give you a batch of numbered capsules which contain various foods.

Ideally, neither she nor you should know what is contained in the capsules. At the end of the test period the 'code' is broken and you and the doctor both find out whether certain foods really were causing the symptoms.

An exclusion diet much used in the United States is the K-P or Feingold diet, which was developed in an effort to help hyperactive children. However, carefully controlled trials have cast doubt on its value.

DRUG ALLERGIES

Unfortunately, allergies to drugs prescribed by doctors are quite common. Both drugs prescribed by a doctor and over-the-counter drugs can cause all sorts of side-effects, but only a minority of these effects are due to an actual allergy.

Common symptoms of a drug allergy include the following:

* skin rashes – If a rash develops after starting medication, always suspect that the drug may be responsible
* wheezing
* fever
* swollen joints

* puffiness of the face

* rarely, complete collapse (*see* **Anaphylaxis**)

If you think you may have a drug allergy, stop using the drug and **call your doctor immediately**.

Among the many drugs which can cause allergic reactions are:

* penicillin in all its forms (this includes ampicillin, amoxycillin and many others)

* aspirin

* anti-histamines (especially when applied to the skin)

* local anaesthetic skin applications.

DUST
(*see* **House dust**)

ECOLOGY – CLINICAL
(*see* **Clinical ecology**)

ECZEMA
This is a very common skin condition. It is important to realise that it is not infectious. It causes a reddish rash, which will be dark if your skin is black or brown) which itches and produces lots of little scales. The skin may also crack and weep, in severe cases.

Eczema most commonly occurs on the knees, elbows, hands and face, but it may turn up almost anywhere. In children under the age of two, the most common sites are the head and trunk.

Unfortunately there is an awful lot of confusion in the way that skin disorders are named and in your part of the world you may well hear eczema referred to as dermatitis. This word simply means inflammation of the skin. One particular form of skin inflammation is contact dermatitis, which may be caused by allergy to something that has been in contact with the skin (*see* **Contact dermatitis**).

There are various types of eczema, but the one we are concerned with here is atopic eczema. The word atopic just means allergic.

Atopic eczema is typified by the following characteristics:

* a strong family tendency to allergy (Mum may have asthma, Dad may have hay fever, and so on)

* a lifelong tendency to react unusually to foreign substances, especially proteins

The condition is often classified by age of onset, as follows:

1 Infantile eczema This is more common in bottle-fed than breast-fed babies, which almost certainly reflects the fact that bottle-fed babies have a sensitivity to the proteins in cow's milk. It often starts between two and four months of age.

The child develops sore-looking patches (though

in fact they do not seem to hurt him), especially round the face, trunk, elbows and knees.

These patches are red (dark in children of African or Asian descent) and have raw areas. There may be cracks, which ooze a little liquid.

Although the appearance of infantile eczema is often quite distressing for the parents, it is important to realise that very often the child is suffering no distress at all. Furthermore, there is a good chance that the eczema will disappear completely within a few years. In other words, there is no particular reason to suppose that he will have eczema all his life.

2 **Childhood eczema** This develops in the toddler years, or slightly later. It most often affects the flexor surfaces of the body – that is, the insides of the joints. The fingers are also commonly affected.

Crusting and cracking are particularly prominent in this age group. There may be weeping from the cracks.

Unfortunately, children with eczema may be subjected to abuse and scorn from school fellows who note the appearance of their skin. It is not unknown for teachers to be ignorant about eczema, and to imply that the condition is contagious – which it isn't – or that it is something to do with dirtiness, which isn't true either. However, many youngsters with this type of eczema do get better by the age of puberty.

3 **Adult eczema** In adult eczema, the skin lesions tend to be thick and crusty with bumps (papules). It is often difficult for the sufferer to stop himself from scratching the itchy places, and this often causes bleeding, and makes the inflammation worse.

In adults, the common sites are the scalp (just where the hair begins), the eyelids, forehead, angle of the mouth, chest elbows, wrists, fingers and knees.

The condition tends to flare up and go down again. Sometimes it may lie dormant for years, and it may go away altogether.

TREATMENT The first principle of treatment is to encourage the child or adult with eczema and help him to understand that the condition is not his fault – or any anybody else's fault either. He should be taught to face the problem of unthinking people who make hurtful remarks, and to be ready to point out that the condition is not infectious, and is nothing to do with lack of cleanliness.

Joining one of the self-help organisations which exist in various countries for eczema is also a good idea.

The second thing to do is to try and identify the allergen. This is not an easy task and you will not find one single allergen which turns out to be the cause of all the symptoms. However it quite often transpires that flare-ups of eczema are caused by specific things, such as a particular shampoo, hair colouring agent or detergent. Avoiding these is very important.

There are other factors which often make eczema worse; they include:

* Excessive use of soap Parents often make the mistake of washing eczematous babies

far too much, because they understandably think that great cleanliness will help

* Excessive use of hot water – this doesn't do eczematous skin any good either

* Stress – although eczema is in itself stressful, it does seem possible that worrying can make the skin worse, so trying to cultivate a calm temperament (easier said than done) may be helpful

* Irritating clothing, with rough bits or sections that press hard on the skin. In general, cool, loose clothing is best

Medication This will have to be determined by your family doctor or, if necessary, dermatologist. But here is a brief guide:

* Dry, scaly patches of eczema can be treated successfully with simple, harmless preparations called emollients.They include such products as aqueous cream and emulsifying ointment. Be cautious about emollients containing lanolin, as these can actually ***cause*** allergic skin reactions. Applications of steroids may help dry and scaly patches *(see* below*),* though these drugs can have unfortunate side-effects. Dry crusts often respond well to keratolytics – these are agents such as salicylic acid that get rid of thickened skin

* Damp, weeping patches may respond to traditional remedies such as potassium permanganate solution, aluminium acete or even calamine lotion. However, these days, it is much more common for steroids to be used

Steroids These are chemical relations of hormones which are produced by the adrenal (suprarenal) glands. For other allergies, such as hay fever or asthma, they are squirted into the nose, inhaled or taken by mouth. In eczema, they are applied to the skin – though very rarely it may be necessary to treat a really bad attack of eczema with oral steroids.

Steroids do work extremely well in many cases of asthma, because of their almost magical ability to 'damp down' inflammation. However, they are extremely powerful drugs, and it is vital that you realise that excessive use (especially of the stronger ones) can be ***very*** harmful indeed. So people with eczema should always be guided by their general practitioners or dermatologists about how much of a steroid they should use rather than just slapping it on and hoping for the best. In particular, be very wary about putting steroids on the face, where permanent damage can easily result.

Side-effects of steroids include:

* serious – sometimes irreversible – thinning of the skin
* permanent red marks on the skin (striae)
* increased hair growth
* inflammation round the mouth, known as perioral dermatitis
* acne
* loss of skin pigment
* flare-up of skin infections

It is also possible for very large doses of skin steroids to be absorbed into the body and have bad effects on the internal organs. This is more likely to happen if the steroid is kept covered by a dressing, which increases its potency.

Generally speaking, mild steroids such as hydrocortisone 1% are relatively safe, but powerful ones such as betamethasone valerate (Betnovate) and clobetasol propionate (Dermovate) are not, and for this reason they must be used strictly in accordance with your doctor's advice.

Alternative therapies These include:

* Exclusion diets It is certainly possible that at least some cases of eczema are caused by food allergies, so there has been much interest – particularly among practitioners of complementary medicine – in the idea of treating the condition with exclusion (elimination) diets. A few years ago it was widely suggested that eliminating dairy products from the diet would help, but careful trials have indicated that while some people with eczema do benefit from this, the majority of people do not. Eggs, chicken and wheat are said to be common provokers of eczema

(*see also* **Diets (exclusion)**)

* Other complementary therapies include Chinese herbs, which have given encouraging results in some patients, and evening primrose oil capsules (Efamol), which are available without prescription

EGGS

Often alleged to be a cause of food allergy. Possible symptoms include skin rashes, wheezing, and swelling of the face and hands.

It is thought to be the protein in the white of the egg that causes the problems; the yolk of eggs does not seem to be very allergenic.

Desensitisation is difficult to achieve. Treatment with oral cromoglycate (Nalcrom) capsules may be helpful. Avoidance of eggs is essential, which is difficult, because they are used in so many things.

(*see also* **Food allergy**)

EPINEPHRINE

The name used in the United States and some other countries for adrenaline (*see* **Adrenaline**).

FISH

Fish, and particularly shellfish, can definitely cause allergies. Symptoms may include rashes, itching, swelling of the mouth and face, and wheezing. In a few cases, the violent and life-threatening reaction of anaphylaxis (*see* **Anaphylaxis**) occurs.

Some people are lucky enough to be allergic to only one species of fish, and can cope with other types. But if you have a serious reaction, and especially anaphylaxis, it is probably best to steer clear of ***all*** fish for the rest of your life. Bear in mind that the name given to a fish on a menu may not always be accurate.

(*see also* **Food allergies**)

FOOD ALLERGIES

Until recently many doctors did not take food allergies seriously and tended to regard the whole idea as rather 'cranky'.

But it is now clear that this was a rather narrow-minded view; after all, allergies can affect many parts of the body, so why not the digestive tract, which is exposed to all sorts of different foodstuffs every day?

There is still have enormous amount to be learned about food allergies, but the common symptoms they produce are thought to include:

* skin rashes (especially urticaria)
* wheezing
* swelling of the hands and face
* possible diarrhoea and tummy-ache

In severe cases, life-threatening collapse (*see* **Anaphylaxis**) may occur. Common food items which may cause problems include peanuts, fish (including shellfish), strawberries, citrus fruits, eggs, wheat and, especially in babies, cow's milk.

The diagnosis of food allergies and the particular food that is causing it is often very difficult. Skin tests are of no use, and testing with exclusion diets (elimination diets) is not easy (*see* **Diet (exclusion)**).

Once the diagnosis is established, it is usually best to try and avoid the offending food altogether. Desensitisation is unlikely to succeed, though clinical ecologists do attempt a form of it.

The anti-allergy drug cromoglycate (Nalcrom), given in capsule form, may help (*see* **Cromoglycate**).

FOOD COLOURINGS AND FLAVOURINGS

(*see* **Additives**)

HAY FEVER

A very common form of allergic rhinitis (*see* **Allergic rhinitis**) – in other words, inflammation of the nose.

Symptoms, which can be very trying indeed, including:

* constant sneezing
* running nose
* a blocked-up feeling
* running, itchy eyes

In addition, a lot of hay fever sufferers feel worn out and cannot produce their best work during attacks. Unfortunately, in many countries the hay fever season coincides with the school/college exam season, so the condition may affect a student's performance – especially if she is taking sedative anti-histamines *(see* below*).*

Hay fever is caused by allergy to pollen, which can be from grasses, flowers, weeds, or trees. Strictly speaking, the word 'hay' refers only to grass, but in practice, all types of allergic nose inflammation caused by pollen are called hay fever.

In the United States, the commonest cause of hay fever is the pollen of ragweed, which grows in all parts of the country, except the north-west, and the area west of the Rockies. Ragweed pollinates between August and October, so the most likely time for hay fever in the United States is the early fall.

In Europe and Australasia, grass pollen is by far the most common cause of hay fever, and the worst time for it is the late spring and early summer. The exact time at which the pollen arrives depends very much on the weather. For instance, hay fever begins several weeks earlier in the south of France than it does in the north of Scotland where it is much cooler.

The pollen is also much higher on dry, fine days. The weather forecasts n many countries, now include an indication of how high the pollen count will be.

DIAGNOSIS The diagnosis of hay fever is usually very obvious, because of its seasonal onset. So with straightforward hay fever, there is absolutely no need to ask your doctor for any special tests. However, if your symptoms arise at rather unusual times of year, when the normal hay fever season is not in full swing – then it may be worth having skin tests to try to find out exactly which kind of pollen is causing the allergy.

If there is any serious doubt as to whether you are really suffering from an allergy, a test on your nasal secretions may reveal certain special 'allergy cells' called eosinophils. Blood tests are only rarely needed.

TREATMENT There are five aspects to the treatment of hay fever:

* avoidance of the allergen (the pollen)
* using antihistamine drugs
* using nasal steroids
* using drugs of the Intal type
* using desensitisation

Avoidance of pollen This should be your first line of defence, before you even think about using drugs. The following measures should help:

* Try to stay indoors on days when the pollen count will be high
* If house windows have to be open, use fine mesh curtains to keep the pollen out
* In cars, keep the windows rolled up
* Stay away from grassy areas or areas where there is ragweed
* When out and about, wear wraparound sunglasses, which help keep pollen out of the eyes
* Consider wearing one of the new anti-pollution smog masks over your mouth and nose

If things get really bad, it is worth thinking about a change of environment Anywhere well away from the plants which are causing the problem should help. Large bodies of water are often free of pollen, so a seaside or lakeside break may do the trick. Indeed even a trip to the local swimming pool will often bring temporary relief.

In the United States it is well worth heading for a desert or mountaintop resort, and almost anywhere west of the Rockies will get you away from ragweed pollen.

Using anti-histamine drugs These are fairly effective in hay fever, but the older ones do tend to make many people very sleepy. The newer ones are less likely to do this, but they can very occasionally have serious side-effects. For full details *see* **Anti-histamines**. A nasal anti-histamine, Rhinolast (azelastine), is used on a small scale.

Using nasal steroids Steroid drugs which are sprayed into the nose have brought great relief to many hay fever sufferers, and in addition, they do not cause drowsiness.

People are often wary of drugs containing steroids, but in fact steroids taken by nose carry very little risk. However, there is a small chance of absorbing enough of them to cause problems with the adrenal (suprarenal) glands, so this type of treatment is usually banned for children under five, and for women in early pregnancy.

The only common side-effects of nasal steroids are itching and dryness of the nose or throat, and possibly nosebleeds. Many people sneeze once or twice after the spray first goes into the nose, but this should be ignored.

The really important thing that hay fever sufferers often do not realise is this: **nasal steroids are no good for treating an actual attack of hay fever**. They have to be used long-term and every day – preferably from the very beginning of the hay fever season until it is completely over.

Common nasal steroid inhalations include Beconase (beclomethasone), Betnesol (betamethasone), Rhinocort (budesonide), Syntaris (flunisolide) and Flixonase (fluticasone). They come in spray or aerosol form, and also in some cases as drops. They should be used between one and four times daily – be guided by your doctor.

Very occasionally, powerful oral (or even injectable) steroids are used in severe cases of hay fever when a person really has an urgent need for relief of symptoms (e.g. when taking an exam). Steroids used in this way carry considerable risks *(see* **Steroids***)*, so doctors do not often suggest this method of treatment in the present day.

Using Intal-type drugs Intal (cromoglycate) is the anti-allergy drug that has been used against asthma to such good effect for three decades. It is not as effective in hay fever, but it can be quite useful. Please remember that it is no help in treating attacks – it has to be used long-term, throughout the hay fever season. It is marketed in various countries as a nasal spray or 'insufflation', under the trade names Rynacrom or Lomusol.

A version for the eyes (eyedrops or ointment) is marketed as Opticrom. Alomide (lodoxamide) and Rapitil (nedocromil) protect the eyes in a similar way. Get full advice from your doctor before using any of these preparations, especially if you wear contact lenses, or are pregnant.

Desensitisation Having desensitising injections before the start of the hay fever season used to be very popular, and it is still practised in the United States. However, although it is quite effective, it has been more or less abandoned in some countries because it carries a risk of serious – and occasionally fatal – collapse.

HERBALISM

A form of alternative medicine that uses herbs to treat allergies (and other conditions too).

There is no reason why you should not try herbal medicine if you wish, but please do make sure that you go to a properly qualified herbalist.

Beware of the attitude which is now widespread that because herbs are 'natural', they cannot be harmful. This is not the case. Traditional herbs such as camomile and golden rod, for example, can cause disastrous allergic reaction in people who have asthma. Herbs used in the Caribbean to treat allergy can give you fatal liver disease.

Traditional Chinese herbs are said to have given good results in eczema and other allergies. But do make sure that any herbal remedy you take does not 'clash' with the treatment your doctor has given you.

HISTAMINE

A 'trouble-making' chemical, released from body cells during allergic reactions (*see* **Allergy**). It is also injected into the body by stinging nettles.

Drugs which counteract the effect of histamine are highly effective (*see* **Anti-histamines**).

HIVES

The name used in North America for urticaria (*see* **Urticaria**).

HOMEOPATHY
This is a form of alternative medicine based on the principle that 'like cures like', and involving the dilution of remedies to extremely low strengths.

Curiously, homeopathy is one branch of complementary medicine that has attracted many doctors, particularly in Great Britain, where most homeopaths are medically qualified.

It is also easy to buy homeopathic remedies at pharmacies in many countries. But personally, I would ***not*** advise treating an allergy yourself.

Homeopaths tend to recommend the following remedies for allergies:

* **Asthma:** nux vomica, aconite, phosphorus
* **Eczema:** sulphur, graphites, mezereum
* **Hay fever:** teucrium, mixed pollen, sabadilla
* **Urticaria:** urtica urens (nettle), sulphur, apis

HOUSE DUST
Many people think they are allergic to dust. But back in the 1960s, research work in Holland showed that it is not the dust itself that so many people are allergic to, but something in it. The 'something' is usually the house dust mite. This tiny creature is present in enormous numbers in many people's homes. Its scientific name is *Dermatophagoides pteronyssimus.*

Dermatophagoides means 'skin-eating', and the mite likes being near human beings, because it eats shed skin cells.

Vast numbers of people are allergic to the house dust mite, or to its droppings, which are breathed into the nose and lungs. This commonly causes a form of allergic rhinitis (inflammation of the nose – *see* **Allergic rhinitis**), but it can also provoke asthma attacks.

It is probable that dust mite allergy has increased a lot in recent years because of the spread of central heating. The mite prefers a temperature of over 25°C (77°F), and a relative humidity of 70 per cent plus. These conditions were rarely obtained in temperate countries before the advent of central heating.

SYMPTOMS AND TREATMENT In addition to causing asthma, the house dust mite can sometimes cause skin irritation. However, the symptoms it most often causes are those of rhinitis:

* sneezing
* running nose
* cracks inside the nose
* blocked-up feeling
* runny eyes
* often, tiredness as a result of attacks

These symptoms are exactly the same as those of hay fever, except that they only occur when the person has been exposed to dust.

Similarly, the treatment of dust mite rhinitis is almost exactly the same as that of hay fever (*see* **Hay fever**), and involves the use of these drugs:

* anti-histamines

* nasal steroids

* Intal-type drugs

Desensitisation against the mite has been tried, but has not proved very successful. What is often successful, however, is avoiding the mite (and its droppings) as far as possible. Good ways to do this include:

* Staying out of lofts and other dusty areas

* Getting rid of 'dust-trap' fixtures, such as drapes, curtains

* Enclosing the sufferer's mattress in a dustproof covering (the mite loves to live in mattresses)

* Vacuuming rooms (especially the bedroom) very thoroughly

* Spraying the bedroom with an anti-dust mite preparation

* Turning the central heating down

* Moving to a non-dusty house, if need be

IgE

Short for immunoglobulin E – the name given to an antibody or, strictly speaking, group of antibodies present at a high level in the blood of many people with allergies. For further details *see* **Allergy**.

It is true to say that IgE is a cause of many

allergies. There is a theory that its original function – way back in the history of the human race – was to help defend our bodies against parasitic infestations.

IMMUNOGLOBULINS

A group of protective substances, or antibodies (*see* **Antibodies**), that help to defend the body against disease. Unfortunately, sometimes there is an abnormality in these defences, and the result is an allergy (*see* **Allergy**).

Immunoglobulins are manufactured by white blood cells called B-lymphocytes.

Immunoglobulins fall into five main categories:

Immunoglobulin G (IgG) makes up about 73 per cent of all immunoglobulins in the body. It gives protection against infections and can cross the placenta (afterbirth) from the mother to the baby, thus giving thus giving the baby some protection against germs.

Immunoglobulin A (IgA) occurs in breast milk and other secretions. It is therefore passed from the mother to her baby, and helps give him further protection against infection. This is one of many reasons why breast milk is preferable to cow's milk. IgA also acts as a general germ fighter around the body.

Immunoglobulin M (IgM) is involved in various protective functions around the body, particularly in attacking germs which get into the bloodstream.

Immunoglobulin D (IgD) is found on the surface of B-lymphocyte white blood cells and is probably involved in body defences.

Immunoglobulin E (IgE) is present at a high level in the blood of allergic people (*see* **IgE**).

INSECT BITES AND STINGS

Note: For stings of bees and wasps, *see* **Bee stings** and **Wasp stings**. For sudden collapse, *see* **Anaphylaxsis**.

Insect bites and stings are extremely common, particularly in the warmer parts of the world and in cooler regions during the summer.

Most bites and stings are no more than minor irritants. But allergic people can sometimes develop quite violent reactions to them, with soreness and swelling extending quite a long way from the site of the original bite.

If this happens, do not scratch; scratching will only make the allergic reaction worse. Put something cold on the affected area and see your doctor; she will probably prescribe anti-histamines (*see* **Anti-histamines**).

Papular urticaria is a bumpy skin eruption, mainly seen in children. It is often intensely itchy, and the child may not be able to stop herself from scratching it. The parents are usually not aware of the original cause: insect bites.

Caterpillar urticaria is a severe eruption of the skin and mouth caused by contact with various species of hairy caterpillars or their windblown parts. Treatment is with anti-histamines (*see* **Anti-histamines**), cold soaks and painkillers.

IONISERS

Ionisers are electrical devices that are supposed to 'soak up' negative electrical charges in the air of a room.

Manufacturers claim that this effect is very good for allergies, such as hay fever and asthma. The evidence for this is at present unconvincing.

IRRITABLE BOWEL SYNDROME (IBS)

IBS is an extremely common condition. Its main symptoms include:

* pain in the tummy
* diarrhoea and/or constipation
* excessive amounts of wind
* a feeling of fullness or bloating

Note: If you have these symptoms, do not diagnose IBS yourself. It is important to see your doctor and have other conditions ruled out.

The causes of IBS are at present unknown, but it does seems likely that in some people at least, some form of allergy will turn out to play a part. As research progesses, far more will become known about this condition.

K–P DIET

Abbreviation for the Kaiser–Permanente diet (*see* **Diet (exclusion)**).

LANOLIN

The fatty extract of sheep's wool, widely used as

a basis for ointments and cosmetics. Unfortunately, a lot of people are allergic to it. The reaction they get in response to lanolin is usually a red (or brown if your skin is dark), bumpy, itchy eruption.

Please note that some popular emollients (soothing agents), including those used to treat eczema (*see* **Eczema**), contain lanolin. They include:

* E45
* zinc cream
* Hewlett's Cream
* Keri
* Massé Breast Cream
* Morhulin
* Morsep
* Sudocrem

If you are allergic to lanolin, you should also avoid products that contain wool fat alcohol. And you will probably also have to avoid lambskin, and possibly wool itself, for a while.

MEDICINES

For allergy to medicines *see* **Drug allergies**.

MIGRAINE

Migraine is a very common condition whose most frequent symptom is blinding pain on one side of the head. As far as we know, it is ***not*** an allergy, but attacks can often be triggered by certain foods, such as oranges, chocolate, nuts, cheese and some red wines. For further information consult your own doctor or your country's migraine association.

MILK

Cow's milk is a common cause of allergy (*see* **Cow's milk allergy**). It is almost impossible for human breast milk to cause an allergy, unless it contains traces of an allergy-producing drug or chemical which the mother has been taking.

If someone is allergic to cow's milk, it should be cut right out of their diet. After babyhood milk is ***not*** an essential for life, although it is a good source of calcium.

But if a child or adult wants to carry on drinking some sort of milk, then it is essential to switch to some 'non-cow' variety. In tropical countries, it is common to drink goat's milk, though this itself can occasionally cause allergy.

In temperate countries, it is more usual to switch to soya milk, which is made from the soya bean, *Soja hispida*. This is the same plant that is used to manufacture soy sauce. Allergy to this milk is most uncommon (*see* **Soya milk**).

MOULDS

A mould is a furry-looking fungal growth. It may drift into the air and be carried into people's noses and lungs. This is particularly likely to happen during the summer months.

In allergic people, the result may be one or both of the following:

* rhinitis (nose inflammation), whose symptoms and treatment are the same as those of hay fever (*see* **Hay fever**)

* asthma (*see* **Asthma**)

There are a number of serious mould infections in which allergy may play a part. They include:

* Cryptococcosis – an infection of the nervous system caused by the species *Cryptococcus neoformans*

* North American blastomycosis – an infection of the lungs and skin, caused by the species *Blastomyces dermatiditis*

* Coccidioidomycosis – an infection of the lungs, lymph nodes and liver caused by the species *Coccidioides immitis*

* Histoplasmosis – a generalised infection caused by the species *Histoplasma capsulatum*.

NUTS

It has become clear in recent years that nuts can be the cause of a very serious type of food allergy. Nuts which commonly cause this problem include peanuts (groundnuts) and pecan nuts.

If a person is allergic to a particular type of nut, eating it can have very serious consequences, resulting in the type of collapse called anaphylaxis (*see* **Anaphylaxis**).

Desensitisation is sometimes attempted, particularly in the United States, but at present the results do not seem encouraging.

If you have this particular allergy, you should avoid the offending nut for the rest of your life. Be particularly wary in cafés and restaurants, where it could easily be contained in pies and vegetarian dishes.

If you have already suffered an attack of anaphylaxis, there is a strong case for carrying a do-it-yourself adrenaline injection kit; ask your doctor for details.

PEAK FLOW METER

Device for doing an important test in asthma (*see* **Asthma**). It measures the maximum flow of air coming out of the patient's mouth during a forceful expiration, in litres per minute. For further details, *see* **Asthma**.

PEANUTS

One of the commoner causes of serious allergic collapse (*see* **Anaphylaxis**). For further details, *see* **Nuts**.

PENICILLIN

One of the most useful of all antibiotics, but unfortunately one of the most likely to cause allergic and sensitivity reactions.

This applies to all forms of penicillin, including Penicillin V, Penbritin (ampicillin), Amoxil (amoxycillin) etc.

The most common form of reaction to penicillin is

a rash. But occasionally, it can cause the serious form of allergic collapse called anaphylaxis (*see* **Anaphylaxis**).

If you are allergic to penicillin, you should carry a note to that effect on your person. Try to ensure that all your medical notes (at a doctor's and/or a hospital) carry a prominent warning that you should not be given penicillin.

(*see also* **Drug allergies**)

PERENNIAL RHINITIS

This means rhinitis (that is, inflammation of the nose) that goes on all the year round. Symptoms are exactly the same as those of hay fever (*see* **Hay fever**), but are present for 12 months of the year.

Sometimes it is possible to identify the allergen which is causing the symptoms – for instance, by skin-testing. In recent years, many cases of perennial rhinitis have turned out to be due to dust mite allergy (*see* **House dust**).

However it is not always possible to identify the provoking factor or factors. In these cases the only solution is drug therapy, as described under the heading **Hay fever**.

POLLEN COUNT

A figure announced daily in many countries during the hay fever season, usually with the weather report and forecast. It gives a good indication of the concentration of pollen grains in the atmosphere.

In general, the pollen count will be high on hot,

dry days. Rainy weather helps to bring it down rapidly.

Knowing the pollen count is a considerable help to most people with hay fever and those who find that their asthma is made worse by pollen.

PRICK TESTS

Allergy tests done by pricking tiny amounts of a solution of an allergen (*see* **Allergens**) into the patient's skin with a needle. Alternatively, the needle may be used to scratch the sufferer's skin slightly.

Although this sounds rather alarming, a prick test is virtually painless, and it is very rare for it to cause any distress to patients.

After the skin is pricked, the area is checked to see if it comes up in a red (or brown) bump, surrounded by a 'flare'. This usually happens within about 15 minutes.

If there is such a reaction then the test is positive, and suggests that the patient is allergic to the substance in question. However, the results of skin tests are not always relevant to the person's illness. For instance, a person may show a positive response to a particular allergen; but that allergen may not be responsible for his asthma or rhinitis.

A rather similar test called a 'patch test' is done with small pieces of materials which are suspected of causing allergy, but which cannot readily be dissolved in a liquid. The material is simply strapped to the patient's forearm and any reaction monitored.

PROCTITIS

Inflammation of the opening of the rectum (the anus), causing redness, soreness and/or itching.

Proctitis can have various causes. It may be due to an allergy or sensitivity – particularly to creams and ointments that have been applied to the bottom. Suppositories may cause similar problems. Occasionally, a drug taken by mouth will produce proctitis, which should clear up as soon as the drug is discontinued.

RHINITIS

Inflammation of the nose, causing:

* sneezing
* snuffling
* a blocked-up feeling
* often, cracks inside the nostrils

Rhinitis is very commonly due to allergy (*see* **Allergic rhinitis**).

SERUM SICKNESS

An unusual type of allergy, sometimes caused by drugs such as antibiotics or aspirin. Blood serum drawn from horses and injected into people to prevent tetanus (lockjaw) used to be a common cause, but is no longer used.

Curiously, serum sickness usually occurs in people who have never previously been exposed to the allergen (*see* **Allergens**).

What happens is that the allergen enters the body in quite a large quantity, and this provokes the body's defences to produce immunoglobulin G-type antibodies (*see under the heading* **Immunoglobulin**).

It appears that there is so much of the antigen (allergen) around that the antibody can react with it there and then, instead of waiting for the next invasion, as is usual in allergic reactions.

The antigen and antibody (together with a body product called complement) form large complexes in the bloodstream. These complexes start to damage parts of the body, including the skin, joints and lymph glands, and possibly the liver.

About seven to ten days after the allergen entered the body, the victim develops an itchy rash, stiff swollen joints, enlarged glands, and possibly protein in the urine.

Although serum sickness can make the sufferer feel extremely unwell for some days, it is usual to make a rapid recovery. Anti-histamines and, if necessary, steroids (*see* **Steroids**) may prove to be helpful.

SKIN TESTING FOR ALLERGY

This is carried out either by prick testing or patch testing (*see* **Prick tests**).

SMOKING

As far as is known, people are not allergic to cigarettes or tobacco. However, any kindof smoking is sheer folly for asthma sufferers (*see* **Asthma**), because it invariably increases the inflammation in the air passages leading to the lungs. In effect, this narrows the air tubes.

Smoking also greatly increases the chances of chest infections, especially as the years go by. Chest infections are a particular threat to asthmatic people, and often trigger off attacks.

In addition, smoking is known to cause lung cancer, and greatly increases the risk of getting various other serious diseases.

To sum up, any person with asthma who decides to smoke is very probably shortening his own life.

Passive smoking If you smoke, your smoke will usually be breathed in by others. This has a bad effect on people with hay fever and other forms of rhinitis, and on people with asthma. It is a particular danger for children who are asthmatic, so it is very important that parents of an asthmatic child do not smoke. It they cannot break the habit, then they should only smoke outside the house.

SOYA MILK

White fluid obtained mainly from the soya bean, *Soja hispide*. It is a useful substitute for 'ordinary' milk in cases of cow's milk allergy.

Types of soya milk currently available include the following products:

* Infasoy, available in powder form. Contains soya protein, carbohydrate (glucose), fat (as vegetable oils), plus vitamins and minerals

* Isomil, available in powder form. Contains soya protein, carbohydrate (corn syrup and sucrose), fat (as soy oil, coconut oil and sunflower oil), plus vitamins and minerals

* Prosobee, available as powder. Contains soya protein, carbohydrate (corn syrup), fat (coconut oil and corn oil), plus vitamins and minerals

* Soya Formula, available as powder. Contains soya protein, carbohydrate (corn syrup), fat (vegetable oils), plus vitamins and minerals

* Wysoy, available as powder. Contains soya protein, carbohydrate (corn syrup), fat (vegetable oils), plus vitamins, minerals and trace elements

Other artificial 'milks' which are not made from soya are available. They include Nutramigen, which is made from casein (cheese-type protein) and other ingredients.

SPERM ALLERGY

Improbable though it sounds, allergy to human seminal fluid (sperm) is said to exist, and was first recorded in medical literature in 1967.

However, it is not a common condition. Only 30 cases have been reported in medical journals over the last three decades.

The symptoms occur in the man's sexual partner. Usually, the woman reports vaginal burning and stinging, beginning a few minutes after ejaculation and persisting for about an hour.

It is necessary to do skin tests to confirm the diagnosis. The antigen (*see* **Antigens**) in question is said to be a protein originating from the male prostate gland.

Sufferers are usually advised to use condoms, unless of course they plan to abstain from intercourse altogether. Anti-histamines (*see* **Anti-histamines**) have also been used. Some doctors have claimed good results from prescribing vaginal application of the anti-allergy drug Intal (*see* **Cromoglycate**).

STEROIDS

Very effective drugs, which are relatives of the steroid hormones produced by the adrenal (suprarenal) glands. Their main effect is to reduce inflammation.

Steroids are extensively used in treating allergy in four main ways:

* on the skin – as described under **Eczema**
* in the nose – as described under **Hay fever**
* by inhalation into the lungs – mainly for asthma *(see* below*)*
* by mouth, in tablet form –, mainly for asthma *(see* below*)*

INHALED STEROIDS FOR ASTHMA These days, people are often worried about using steroids, because they fear their side-effects. But it is important to realise that the inhaled steroids that are used in asthma produce very few serious ill-effects, and do not share the same dangers as oral steroids *(see* below*)*. However, no steroid is without the risk of side-effects, even when inhaled. Recent research has shown that it is possible they might have an effect in making bones thinner, though this has not been a problem so far. They can also cause hoarseness and (in larger doses) thrush infection in the throat or mouth. Washing the mouth out after use can help prevent this.

Mode of use It is vitally important to realise that inhaled steroids must be used ***regularly*** and ***as prescribed*** if they are to work. Taking them occasionally is useless, and they are of no real value in an actual attack. It takes up to a week before their benefit is felt.

Steroids are inhaled from special devices *(see* **Asthma***)* and work best through a spacer, which is designed to get more of the steroid into the lungs, leaving less 'wasted' in the mouth and throat. Special suspensions of steroids which can be inhaled very efficiently from a nebuliser are now available.

Inhaled steroid products include:

* beclomethasone dipropionate (Becotide, AeroBec, Becodisks, etc.
* budesonide (Pulmicort)
* fluticasone propionate (Flixotide)

ORAL STEROIDS Steroids taken by mouth are entirely different, because they spread through the body and can produce all sorts of unwanted effects. For this reason, doctors try to confine their use mainly to emergencies – when they are frequently life-saving.

Possible side-effects experienced when taking steroid tablets include:

* growth stunting in children
* raised blood pressure (hypertension)
* osteoporosis (thinned bones)
* diabetes
* stomach ulcers

* muscle wasting

* excitement and mental disturbances

* acne

* Cushing's syndrome

* skin damage

*spread of infections

From this formidable list, you can see that you should never take steroid pills casually, but only use them as your doctor advises. However, your doctor may give you with a small emergency supply to be taken if symptoms get appreciably worse or if your peak expiratory flow' (*see* **Peak flow meter** and **Asthma**) seems to be deteriorating to a dangerously low level. If you start yourself on one of these courses, always let your doctor know, and go and see her for a checkup as soon as possible.

Please note that oral steroids must ***not*** be stopped suddenly. They must always be 'tailed off' over a period of several days.

If you are on oral steroids, you should carry a special 'steroid card' on your person at all times in case you are involved in an accident or taken to hospital.

Oral steroid preparations include:

* prednisolone (Prednisol, Precortisyl Forte)

* prednisone (Decortisyl)

* betamethasone (Betnelan, Betnesol)

* dexamethasone (Decadron)

INJECTABLES Steroids can also be given by injection, though this is almost always done by a doctor, rather than the asthmatic patient herself. An injection of steroid is quite often life-saving if given during a really bad attack.

Injections of a steroid-related drug, ACTH, are still self-administered by patients in some parts of the world for non-emergency treatment of asthma.

STICKING PLASTER

Allergy or sensitivity to sticking plaster is extremely common. It is easy to diagnose, because a couple of days after putting the plaster on, the person comes out in a rash which exactly matches the shape of the plaster.

If you suffer from this allergy, the best thing to do is to use only hypo-allergenic plasters, which are now quite widely available If really necessary, a bad eruption can be treated with oral anti-histamines (*see* **Anti-histamines**).

STRAWBERRIES

This fruit is a common cause of food allergy (*see* **Food allergies)**. The most common symptom is a rash, but it has also been suggested that strawberries may cause dizziness. Very occasionally anaphylaxis (*see* **Anaphylaxis**) may occur.

Unfortunately, desensitisation is unlikely to be a practical possibility for dealing with this allergy.

(*see also* **Urticaria** for more information)

STRESS

Until recently, doctors tended to hold the view that people with allergies were rather tense individuals, and that therefore allergies were partly caused (or at least made worse) by stress.

In fact, vast numbers of people with allergies are not particularly stressed at all. And even when they are rather fraught individuals, it could well be that the allergy is contributing to the tension.

Nonetheless, if you have a severe allergy it does seem sensible to try to avoid strain and worry as much as possible, though this may be difficult.

TOTAL ALLERGY SYNDROME

In the last 20 years or so, there has been an extraordinary proliferation of media reports about people who are alleged to be allergic to everything. It is claimed that they collapse and become seriously ill when they are exposed to absolutely anything at all, except totally 'pure' items such as oxygen and water which has been distilled many times over.

One can only have sympathy for such people, who are obviously living the most terrible existence. However, orthodox doctors who specialise in allergy will tell you that these claims are completely without foundation, no matter how sincerely the patient may believe in them.

Regrettably, there are doctors –especially in the United States – who also believe in 'total allergy', and who will arrange improbable therapies in special units which are designed to keep out all possible outside 'influences'. One patient collapsed when a TV microphone was allowed into her secure unit; it was then alleged that she was allergic to the microphone.

While 'total allergy syndrome' sufferers may well have ***some*** allergies, it seems likely that their main problems are linked with such conditions as over-breathing (hyperventilation). This is a common cause of collapse in people who are upset and frightened.

'TWENTIETH CENTURY ALLERGY'

This is a newspaper term for total allergy syndrome (*see* above). Presumably in the year 2001 it will be changed to 'twenty-first century allergy syndrome'.

URTICARIA

A very common allergic skin condition, known in the United States and elsewhere as 'hives'. It produces a red, raised rash which is quite similar in appearance to extensive nettle stings – in some parts of the world urticaria is called 'nettle rash'.

The bumps on the skin are referred to as 'wheals' – an unusual medical word, not to be confused with 'weals', which are marks caused by a whip.

The wheals are usually pale in the middle, and red round the edges. They are accompanied by itching sensations.

Often the cause of urticaria cannot be found, but it is thought that in most cases it is due to release of the 'allergy chemical', histamine (*see* **Histamine**). Where a cause can be identified, it is usually one of the following:

* food – especially strawberries, shellfish, eggs or pork
* drugs – especially aspirin and penicillins
* parasites, such as worms – mainly in tropical countries

Some types of urticaria clear up rapidly on their own, and never return. Others keep coming back whenever the sufferer is exposed to the allergen, so if you know that strawberries bring you out in a rash, you should make every effort to avoid them in the future.

Mild attacks of urticaria should be left to subside. More troublesome ones are treated with anti-histamines (*see* **Anti-histamines**). In severe cases (giant urticaria) treatment with powerful steroid drugs may be needed (*see* **Steroids**).

Desensitisation has not proved very successful. Fortunately, some do just seem to get over a tendency to urticaria, for no obvious reason.

For papular urticaria and caterpillar urticaria, *see* **Insect bites and stings**.

Urticaria pigmentosa is a distinct condition and bears no apparent relation to allergy.

WASHING POWDERS (*see* **Detergents**)

WASP STINGS

For most people, wasp stings are no more than a painful nuisance. All you need to do is put on a cold, wet dressing and wait for the pain to go away. If really necessary, you can take a painkiller such as aspirin or paracetamol.

However, in some allergic people a wasp sting may cause the terrifying collapse called anaphylaxis (*see* **Anaphylaxis**). If this happens, the victim should be rushed to hospital straight away and those with him should be prepared to give the kiss of life and/or heart massage.

If you have had a previous collapse of this sort, you should go out of your way to avoid wasps.

Wear an insect repellent on your skin when you go outside in summer. Be extremely wary about where you put your hands, especially when there is jam or some other wasp attractant around. You should also take great care to look at any outdoor drink – especially sweet ones – before putting it to your lips.

Previous victims of anaphylaxis may well wish to obtain a do-it-yourself adrenaline injection kit; ask your doctor for details.

Desensitisation against wasp venom is available, but cannot be guaranteed to give total protection.

YEAST ALLERGY

Yeasts often attack the body – especially candida (monilia), the organism which causes vaginal thrush in women and thrush in babies' mouths.

The popular press often claims that celebrities are suffering from 'yeast allergies', but whether it is really possible to be allergic to a yeast is not yet clear.

Yeasts are usually treated successfully with drugs such as Canesten (clotrimazole).

APPENDIX

Drugs Used Against Allergies

Acrivastine

A fairly non-sedating anti-histamine (*see*: **anti-histamines**) used in hay fever and urticaria. This relatively new drug should be avoided by people who suffer from kidney problems.

Adrenaline

Known in the US and many other countries as 'epinephrine', this drug is enormously useful in the treatment of life-threatening allergic conditions, such as anaphylactic shock. It has to be given by injection.

Antazoline

Drug used against eye allergies, particularly allergic conjunctivitis. Administered as eye drops, often mixed with other drugs such as xylometezoline, anatazoline is an anti-histamine, but the eye drops do not cause sedation.

Astemizole

Non-sedative anti-histamine, used against urticaria and hay fever. Do not take during pregnancy. Women of child-bearing age should use contraception while taking this drug and for several weeks afterwards. Do NOT combine with other medication.

Azatadine

Sedative anti-histamine, useful in hay fever, urticaria and other allergies. Co-ordination and the ability to perform skilled tasks will be impaired. Do not take alcohol while on azatadine.

Azelastine

Anti-histamine used in nasal sprays for allergic rhinitis, when it should not cause sedation. Less effective than steroid nose sprays.

Beclomethasone

Steroid agent, used against allergic rhinitis as a nasal spray, against asthma in inhaler form; and against severe eczema as a cream or ointment.

Betamethasone

Another steroid agent, used in tablets for suppressing serious allergies, in creams or ointments for skin allergies; and in drops for inflammations of the eyes, ear and nose.

Budesonide

Steroid agent, used in inhaler form against asthma; also as a cream or ointment against allergic skin disorders; and also in aerosol or spray form against allergic rhinitis.

Cetirizine

A fairly new and relatively non-sedating

anti-histamine drug. Useful against hay fever and other allergies. For fuller details, seek the advice of your physician or pharmacist.

Chlorpheniramine

Long-established traditional anti-histamine, much used against hay fever, skin allergies and anaphylactic reactions. Chlorphenicamine is VERY sedative. Do not drive or undertake tasks requiring co-ordination. Do not take alcohol.

Cinnarizine

An anti-histamine used in the treatment of allergic reactions, and also in Ménière's disease. Highly sedative, and may cause skin problems, and other side-effects.

Cromoglycate

Also known as 'sodium cromoglycate' or as 'disodium cromoglycate', this drug is a useful preventive against allergic reactions. It has to be taken regularly, since it is of no use in the treatment of actual attacks.

Cyclizine

Anti-histamine, occasionally used in the treatment of allergy, but more often in the therapy of nausea and travel sickness. Sedative. Do not drive, do not take alcohol.

Cyproheptadine

Anti-histamine, used particularly against allergic rhinitis and urticaria. May cause weight gain. Sedative in effect. Do not drive or operate machinery. Do not drink alcohol.

Dexamethasone

A potent steroid, used in the suppression of severe allergic disorders. For full details of potential side effects and essential precautions, consult your physician. Also available (through prescription only) as drops for the treatment of eye allergies.

Dimenhytdrate

Anti-histamine used to treat allergies in some parts of the world, but more often employed against motion sickness and vertigo. Sedative. Do not drive, operate machinery or drink alcohol.

Diphenhydramine

Anti-histamine, useful against hay fever and other allergies. Highly sedative (in fact, often prescribed as a sleeping pill), so do not drive or operate machinery. Do not drink alcohol.

Disodium cromoglycate

See **Cromoglycate**, *above.*

Doxylamine

Anti-histamine, widely used as an ingredient in cough medicines and decongestant preparations – though it will only be of value if there is an allergic component in the disorder. Sedative. Do not drink alcohol, drive or operate machinery.

Epinephrine *See* **Adrenaline**, *above.*

Flunisolide

Steroid used as an aqueous nasal spray to treat hay fever and other forms of allergic rhinitis. May cause transient sneezing when first used.

Fluticasone

Another steroid, used as an aqueous nasal spray in treating various forms of allergic rhinitis. Like other steroid nasal sprays, it may cause minor episodes of sneezing when first used.

Hydrocortisone

Steroid. Milder than many other steroid preparations, but must nonetheless be used with caution. Available in various forms (pills, eye drops, creams, ointments, etc.). A fairly weak (17) hydrocortisone cream is available without prescription in many parts of the world for treatment of skin allergies. Do not use on the FACE, it case it causes permanent damage.

Hydroxyzine

Anti-histamine mainly used when allergies cause itching of the skin. This sedative is also prescribed in cases of anxiety. Do not drive or operate machinery, do not take alcohol.

Ketotifen

An anti-histamine drug which has been used with variable effectiveness in asthma. Believed to have an action rather like that of cromoglycate (*see above*). Sedative. Do not drive or drink. Do not use with oral anti-diabetic drugs.

Lodoxamide

Anti-inflammatory drug used in the form of drops for eye allergies, such as allergic conjunctivitis. May cause a slight, transient stinging sensation.

Loratadine

Relatively non-sedative anti-histamine drug, used in the treatment of various allergies, including allergic rhinitis and urticaria. At present, loratadine should not be used during pregnancy.

Mequitazine

Anti-histamine, useful in treating hay fever and some other allergies. Sedative, so do not drink alcohol or drive or operate machinery. Not for children under 12 at present.

Methylprednisolone

Steroid drug which suppresses inflammation in various allergic disorders. Available as tablets or injection, and also as a cream for the treatment of eczema. For full details of side-effects and precautions, consult your doctor.

Nedocromil

An anti-asthma drug, believed to have a similar action to that of cromoglycate (*see* **Cromoglycate**, *above*). Taken via an aerosol. Used as a preventative – not for the treatment of acute attacks. May cause headache or nausea

Oxatomide

Anti-histamine used to relieve hay fever, food allergy and urticaria. It has sedative effects, so do not drive, operate machinery or drink alcohol. Higher doses may cause weight gain.

Phenindamine

Sedative anti-histamine used to treat hay fever and urticaria. Do not drive or operate machinery. Do not drink alcohol.

Pheniramine

Sedative anti-histamine used against allergic rhinitis and skin allergies. Also included in certain cough medicines, though there is little point in this unless the cough has an allergic component. Do not combine with alcohol. Do not drive or operate machinery.

Prednisolone

Powerful steroid used (as tablets or injections) to suppress inflammation in allergic disorders. Valuable in severe asthma. For full details of side-effects and precautions, consult your physician. Prednisolone is also available in the form of drops, for allergies of the eye or ear.

Prednisone

Powerful steroid, very similar in nature to **prednisolone** (*see above*).

Promethazine

Widely used anti-histamine especially good for hay fever and anaphylactic shock. Also included in many cough and decongestant preparations which are on sale to the public. Strong sedative effects. Do not drive or operate machinery. Do not take alcohol.

Sodium cromoglycate

See **Cromoglycate**, *above.*

Steroids

Strong anti-inflammatory drugs, many of which are useful against allergies. They can have many side-effects, and it can be dangerous to take them other than as prescribed. Always follow your own doctor's advice to the letter. If you are on oral steroids (ie tablets by mouth), you should carry a card which says so.

Terfenadine
Relatively non-sedating anti-histamine. Useful in allergic rhinitis, including hay fever. Occasionally causes heart problems in high doses, so never exceed the stated dose. Never take any other drug with terfenadine, unless your doctor says it is safe to do so.

Triamcinolone
Strong steroid drug used (by injection or in table form) in severe allergies. For more information about side-effects and precautions, take your doctor's advice. Triamcinolone is also available in cream or ointment form for severe skin allergies.

Trimeprazine
Anti-histamine, widely used against urticaria and also any type of itching caused by an allergy. Sedative, so do not drive or operate machinery. Avoid alcohol.

Triprolidine
Anti-histamine used in urticaria and hay fever. Sedative, so do not drive or operate machinery. Do not take alcohol. Triprolidine is contained in various preparations for coughs, but is unlikely to help unless the cough has an allergic basis.